Cancer is Your Choice

Frederick Mickel Huck

authorHOUSE®

AuthorHouse™
1663 Liberty Drive
Bloomington, IN 47403
www.authorhouse.com
Phone: 1-800-839-8640

First published by AuthorHouse 8/21/2009

ISBN: 978-1-4490-0762-1 (sc)

Library of Congress Control Number: 2009907094

Printed in the United States of America
Bloomington, Indiana

This book is printed on acid-free paper.

This book is dedicated to:

ROBERT E MENZIE

INEZ A MENZIE

DONALD W HUCK

AURA V HUCK

DR EDE KOENIG

Special thanks to:

SANDRA V MOONEY

MATTHEW F MOONEY

ANGIE INGERSOLL

About the Book

My purpose in writing this book is to achieve one goal, to explain the cause of cancer in a way that can be easily understood. I have applied common sense and used research to explain why cancer exists and why it continues at epidemic levels. I have explained why the present oncology protocol does not work, and what can be done if one is diagnosed with cancer, how to prevent cancer without drugs or medical advice. I have also explained why the medical system, including cancer charities, prosper financially and owe their financial interest to cancer. In spite of all the promises that have been made by the drug companies, there are not any drugs that can rid the body of cancer.

Improper nutrition is the primary cause of cancer. Not the lack of expensive drugs. The huge medical establishment has a vested interest to maintain cancer and to keep things as they are. None of the current oncology protocols or methods work, yet the medical establishment continues to discredit natural and historical proven methods. People have been fooled for a long time about cancer treatments. The medical establishment works only on the symptoms of cancer, not the causes; this explains why cancer deaths are not decreasing but in fact are going up. If a patient is told that he is in remission he is still sick; because the cancer is still present and will not go away. Cancer can not exist if understood. Mistreating the body will cause the body not to function properly. I have endeavored to explain how cancer can be reversed by our own body and how your body will respond in a manner consistent with a healthy life. In this book there are many common sense suggestions and delicious recipes that will not promote but prevent cancer.

After all cancer is your choice.

The Children

It is the responsibility of adults to teach proper nutrition by examples to children. However that responsibility is not being achieved. Proper nutrition does not promote cancer but poor nutrition does. Good nutrition has the proper nutrients, that the human body needs for growth, repairs, and rebuilding. Poor nutrition is the primary cause of cancer, and chemicals placed in the body is the secondary cause of cancer. Before children are born they are consuming food in the womb of their mother. If the mother is using proper nutrition the unborn child is too. After the birth of a child it is extremely important to provide proper food for the baby, so he will have a disease free life and a fully functioning body.

It is the opinion of this author that it is wrong and immoral to raise unhealthy and sick children. Especially, when we have the knowledge and ability to prevent and eliminate cancer through proper nutrition. In this book you will find some great recipes that are examples of good food that will bring the reader closer to nature and radiant health and away from disease and cancer. If the reader uses the recipes that are included in this book, he will have a more complete life that is free from pain, suffering, an early death and or financial ruin. Also this book will give your children a much better start in life. In life we often come across people whom I call friendly enemies, friends who unknowingly give bad advice. We should all be on the lookout for these "enemies", if they encourage us to do any of the following unhealthy things: radiation, chemo therapy, surgery, and or drugs, eating unhealthy, eating junk foods, using any available oils, sunlamps, sun screens, sun blockers, waiting for new drugs, donating money for cancer research, any health organizations, and or continuing to get check ups to see if cancer has shown up yet. What to do to prevent cancer? I strongly suggest reading "Weight Loss Solutions Your Body Will Accept" and follow it closely. Spend extra time on setting up the pantry, followed through on restaurant test dos and don'ts recipes, colon hydro therapy, and locate a naturalpathic doctor who will work with you. By doing this your body may not be stricken with cancer.

What to do if diagnosed with cancer?

Cancer is a malfunction in the body which can be reversed. Cancer is caused by abusing the body over many years, but cancer is preventable. Start by eating clean food and clean your body with hydro therapy. Associate yourself with a naturalpathic doctor. Once this is done your immune system will correct the body's deficiencies, and will start to correct and repair itself. What goes in the body and on the body are the key reversals to cancer problems. After this process is completed one needs to maintain this new life style. It has been increasingly common to hear that a famous person or celebrity has announced that they have cancer, or even one of your friends or family members may have been diagnosed with cancer. The results are all the same. They are prescribed drugs, then the pain, suffering, and finally death.

Cancer is diagnosed in every city everyday in this country, but yet the suggested treatment is a waste of time and money because the treatment does not work. The best treatment for cancer is do not abuse your body by eating the wrong foods. You will not get cancer if you eat the right foods.

The Medical Doctors Role in Your Life

Do not blame doctors, blame the system. Doctors are doing what they are taught in medical school, and be aware they prosper economically from those established methods that they practice. However it does not take too long to know and to see that most of the therapies do not work. Doctors do not cure cancer but they do prosper economically with their worthless procedures.

Cancer Therapies

Most every thinking person would rather be involved in prevention and not ever be stricken with cancer.

Drugs

All drugs are toxic to the body and all have side effects. If one continues to take drugs their body will malfunction. Just ask any doctor to list and explain all the side effects to any drugs that are on the market today. These drugs are poison, toxic, and possibly deadly for you.

Cutting

Any surgery to the body affects the entire body and may cause more harm than good. Surgery is not the cause of cancer; it is a side effect and it can not be the solution.

Radiation

The human body responses and reactions to radiation can vary greatly. It may include loss of hair, skin color can change, the therapy destroys parts of the body, and interferes and lowers the body's natural defense and immune system. All therapies will hurt the human body and it will still have cancer. If doctors claim the cancer is in remission one still may have cancer.

It is the hope of this author that doctors will sooner rather than later promote good food, a clean body, good advice, and a drug free healthy environment, as their role in our lives.

The naturalpathic doctors role in your life.

A relationship should be established and developed for guidance in nutrition and natural remedies. This includes knowledge and direction in herbal therapies when necessary. Your naturalpathic doctor is very well educated in how the human body functions and of course what causes it to malfunction , and will advise their patients to never take any drugs or have any operations unless it is a rare emergency. If drugs are involved in such an event, colon therapy can be given to remove the drug residue from the body. With this kind of relationship and guidance you, your family, and friends will certainly be in good health.

Parasites and Worms

To achieve a long and healthy life it is important to eat nutritional foods, which do not contain parasites or worms as they can cause blockage in the intestines, inflame and even destroy tissue, cause heart problems, increase weight, produce asthmatic symptoms, stomach aches, colitis, liver problems, and eye problems due to larva around the eyes, skin eruptions, depression, energy loss, anemia and a lowered immune system.

Worms and parasites can invade your body in many ways including but not limited to tap water, animal, contact with people, overseas travel, going barefoot and unsanitary conditions.

Your body can be host for many unwanted guest. First of all there are thousands of parasites, and approximately two hundred to three hundred worms that can invade the human body. Some are up to forty feet long (tapeworm). The most popular worms are hook worms, pinworms, inchworms, black worms, round worms (they produce over 200,000 eggs per day) white worms, fish worms, whip worms, spider worms, fuzz worms, stick pin worms, giardia lambia are found in household drinking water and are chlorine resistant, one thousand can fit on the head of a pin. There are different kinds of tapeworms. The beef tapeworm averages 13 to 39 feet long. The tapeworms that come from fish are the largest and can produce one million eggs per day. Each person has approximately 30 to 50 pounds of parasites in his body at any one time

For a healthy body it is very important that all the worms, toxins, parasites, and bad bacteria be eliminated from ones body. Doctors are not usually the best source to consult on this subject, as their education on the entire topic of worms and parasites consists of one college microbiology class. It is a fact that **intestinal parasites** and worms are not understood and are poorly diagnosed. Working with symptoms does not work very well. The cause of a problem should be examined very carefully. By definition parasites and worms are at an epidemic level. Parasites , worms, toxins and bacteria cause many problems in the **human body**. The resources are available to eliminate parasites, toxins, and bad bacteria through proper nutrition and can stop the body from being a host.

WATER PICK AND ORAL IRRIGATOR

I see a major improvement in the quality of my life, by using proper oral hygiene. A water pick is extremely beneficial to good oral hygiene. This amazing device should be used two to three times a day along with brushing with peppermint oil and ozone water. The long term benefits will be less dental expenses, and increase in your quality of life, and decrease in contacting cancer.

The immune system can be lowered by gum disease, bacteria, tooth decay, tooth sensitivity, gum recession, and tooth loss. Problems with oral hygiene can effect the entire body. The water pick is also a great way to eliminate major tooth and bone problems. This is another good reason to add this equipment to your pantry list.

HYPERBARIC OXYGEN THERAPY

What is this relationship to the body with cancer? This equipment or chamber is a bell shaped dome and is very small. There is just enough room for two people to sit inside. The equipment was used historically for divers with the bends, using high pressure oxygen to force nitrogen out of the blood system. This procedure was common to see in old movies. One or two people would sit in an upright position for forty five minutes to an hour. There are newer models where a person will lie down and receive the same benefits. In either system the person breaths pure oxygen at a pressure above normal atmospheric pressure. This procedure will also increase the oxygen to the entire body. The following are just some of the benefits of hyperbaric therapy: fights infections, wounds, anemia, kills bacteria, prevents strokes, skin damage, prevents lesions due to burns, and sores. In addition to moving past a crisis stage such as a person with cancer, with more white cells than red blood cells. This extra oxygen can help make the difference between life and death. This therapy can be used for any body malfunction. It is not limited to divers coming up too fast from water. The knowledge of this therapy is being used more and more and in the future will increase in popularity with positive results. It is recommended to go through this procedure before and after a cleansing of your body. There are many benefits to this hyperbaric oxygen therapy and it is recommended to check with your naturalpathic doctor before beginning treatment.

COLON THERAPY

I will now attempt to answer the following questions:
1. How to get colon therapy?
2. Where to go?
3. How often?
4. Does colon therapy have a history?
5. Why is it not widely known?

A colon therapist is also known as an inner bath hydro therapist who is trained and certified in anatomy, physiology, hygiene sanitation, massage ethics, and the technical working of the equipment. These practitioners are not hard to find. One can consult a naturalpathic doctor for a referral to a colon therapist.

Colon therapy is a type of bath for the colon and is considered as a necessity, that the human body requires. If done properly the colon bath will clean and wash both the large and small intestine. It requires special equipment that uses air pressure and purified water that breaks up hard impactions, waste, fecal material, worms, bacteria, toxins, and parasites, that is in the walls of large and small intestines. The colon becomes dirty by eating the wrong types of foods, unclean fruits and vegetables, and animal products. All animal products have the following in common: poisons, toxins, parasites, worms, and bacteria. Junk food is overly processed, lacks fiber, is concentrated, has sugar, oils, chemicals, and drugs. This is what causes the colon to become dirty and causes other parts of the body to not work properly. If a person has caused his colon to become dirty and causes other parts of the body to not work properly. If a person has caused his colon to become dirty he should undergo colon therapy and never allow the colon to become dirty again. To clean out the intestines it is recommended six one hour sessions (one per day) and then consult your naturalpathic doctor for advice on how many more sessions may be needed.

Early Egyptians, Greeks, and other ancient people used a variety of methods to wash and clean the colon. Often the procedures were used when sickness, illness, and even body injuries were present. Colds, flu, and other problems would be prevented or less severe utilizing colon cleansing. Today with the development of sophisticated colonic irrigation machines and with results being seen, come an interest to learn more about colon health. More people are turning to natural methods in taking control of their health. But beware! The American medical community has and is trying to suppress information on colon therapy. As more people are learning about colon therapy, the information process and costs are becoming more readily available as the market grows. It is exciting to be part of a drugless therapy that is being redefined and improved upon to give the human race a chance for better health and a better quality of life. Use common sense and do not listen to anyone who wants to promote methods that do not work. In my reference pages are included a small group of noted scientists and researchers who are not sponsored by drug companies. These researchers did not receive the attention that they deserved, because they were not funded by companies that are solely in the business to make money. When common sense is applied to a cancer problem it can be understood easily, because one will know what works without having to go through all the medical confusion. With proper information one can see and avoid cancer problems. It is obvious that cancer therapies do not work. The medical system of doctors, hospitals, pharmaceutics, and the entire medical system have a large financial stake in fake medical cures because their income depends on cancer patients. Having no cancer patients means a loss of income to all those involved in the system.

CONCLUSION

I urge everyone to do their own research, as I have, to avoid cancer. Knowing the cause of cancer and doing what it takes to eliminate it will prevent one from getting cancer. That's all it takes. Avoid the present therapies that most doctors use for they do not work. Just treating the symptoms and not the causes absolutely makes no sense. If one desires a long life without pain, suffering, and large medical bill you need to follow my advice. Take a proactive care approach for your well being, and do not mistreat your body and hope that it will recover by itself. The human body will malfunction if a correction is not made. Within this book are some delicious food recipes. This food is healthy and will not harm the body; instead it will promote radiant health which you deserve. This book in its entirety is dedicated to those who lost their lives to a cancer hoax, implemented by the medical system; and for those who will prevent or make the change not to be part of a cancer farce. It is your body -- get it cleaned and never mistreat it again. Cancer is your choice.

About the Author

The early death of my father is responsible for my journey into researching a healthy life style through proper nutrition. The lung cancer that killed my father was preventable. It is my goal to inform others so that no one else has to witness a loved one die a death needlessly. I mistakenly thought that there was only thirteen days of warning for my father's condition. He entered the hospital July the tenth and was deceased on July twenty third. The warnings were there but ignored for years. The warnings were persistent coughing, noticeable aging of the body, more doctor visits, drugs, and a sick like appearance. I have little trust in the medical system. It is a very large business that exists for outrageous profits. It receives one seventh of the country's GNP (Gross National Product) and only treats symptoms, not the root causes which is prevention. Remember that an ounce of prevention is worth a pound of cure.

Prevention is the only way to achieve a healthy life. For those who have already been diagnosed with cancer, I am going to provide you with information on how to live a higher quality of life without cancer.

Guide 14 Days

The purpose of this fourteen day meal plan is to illustrate that starvation does not exist when following the plan. Instead of listing the fruit on a daily log everyday, I just list here approximately what was eaten.

For the last two years, I have reversed my two meals. The larger was consumed first and the second is mostly raw. Prior to eating breakfast, generally a half an hour after I wake, I drink a quart of warm water with two teaspoons of lemon juice, one tablespoon of inland sea water, and one tablespoon of silver mineral water. I consume approximately five pounds of fruit daily, and the fruit varies according to the seasons of the year.

The fourteen days are very similar (fruit meal) and they are three different colors of apples, twelve cherries, one nectarine, one mango, one slice of pineapple, one slice of cantaloupe, eight green grapes, one apricot, and one peach,. In addition I also eat eight raw Brazil nuts, six apricot nuts, one teaspoon of sunflower seeds, one teaspoon of pumpkin seeds, two capsules of calcium, two capsules of magnesium. For dinner, I usually have a salad which consists of: red or green head lettuce three radishes cut small one long green, onion cut small one third of a carrot, cut small one half of avocado one half of celery stalk, cut small six tablespoons of lemon juice approximately one tablespoon or more of Braggs Ammino up to twelve ounces or more of two different kinds of Hot Sauce bread, or crackers, or corn tortillas

Please do not copy or give away any material, not just because it is copyright protected material, but doing this will interfere with my program of feeding and educating the unhealthy. All book proceeds as of 2008 have gone into this program. Instead my wish is that you do share your cooking with friends, family, and strangers.

Questions, concerns, and suggestions are welcome:
Phone 559 435 4069

14 Days of Meals

Day 1

Breakfast: Fruit,

Raw Nuts

Dinner: Salad,

2 stuffed bell peppers,

6 ounces of Black Eyed Pea-Rice

Crackers

Dessert: One fourth pound of Walnut Square Cookies

Day 2

Breakfast: Fruit,

                    Raw Nuts

Dinner: Salad,

                    12 ounces of Chinese Soup

                    12 ounces of Havenero Baked Rice

                    6 ounces of Cajun roasted nut mix

                    Cornbread

Dessert: One fourth pound RHI carob and roma oatmeal cookies

Day 3

Breakfast: Fruit,

                 Raw Nuts

Dinner: Salad,

                 Pot pie

                 6 ounces of Texan Rice

                 Crackers

Dessert: One fourth pound of Carob Pie

Day 4

Breakfast: Fruit,

               Raw Nuts

Dinner: Salad,

               12 ounces of Black eyes peas

               12 ounces of Bell Pepper Rice

               Soymilk Cornbread

Dessert: One fourth pound of Carob Doughnuts

Day 5

Breakfast: Fruit,

Raw Nuts

Dinner: Salad,

Roast

6 ounces of Spanish rice

Bread

Dessert: One fourth pound of Nut Pie

Day 6
Breakfast: Fruit,

Raw Nuts

Dinner: Salad,

12 ounces of Pan Fried Noodles

12 ounces of Chinese Rice

Crackers

Dessert: Carob cookies

Day 7

Breakfast: Fruit,

                Raw Nuts

Dinner: Salad,

                4 pocket pizzas

                Crackers

Dessert: One fourth pound of pineapple pie

Day 8

Breakfast: Fruit,

Raw Nuts

Dinner: Salad,

2 Tamales

12 ounces of Spanish rice

Bread

Dessert: One fourth pound of Papaya walnut cookies

Day 9

Breakfast: Fruit,

             Raw Nuts

Dinner: Salad,

             12 ounces of Lentils

             12 ounces of Baked Brown Rice

             Corn tortillas

Dessert: One fourth pound of Maple Syrup cookies

Day 10

Breakfast: Fruit,

Raw Nuts

Dinner: Salad,

Pasta

Crackers

Dessert: Lemon Pineapple Ice cream

Day 11
Breakfast: Fruit,

               Raw Nuts

Dinner: Salad,

               4 large baked potatoes with cheese sauce

               6 ounces of Bell Pepper Rice

               Crackers

Dessert: One fourth pound of Pineapple face cookies

Day 12

Breakfast: Fruit,

Raw Nuts

Dinner: 2 Taco Salads

Dessert: Pineapple cookies

Day 13

Breakfast: Fruit,

Raw Nuts

Dinner: Salad,

3 Beerocks

Corn tortillas

Dessert: Carob pastry

Day 14
Breakfast: Fruit,

Raw Nuts

Dinner: Salad

3 Egg Rolls

6 ounces of Chinese Rice

2 slices of Garlic bread

Dessert: One fourth pound of coffee cake

Recipe 94 ─────────────────────

Pot Pies

Place the following in a large pan and boil for 15 minutes on low:

    One half cup of peas
    One half cup of shredded carrots
    One onion cut small
    One teaspoon of bio-salt
    One can of green olives, each cut in half
    One stalk of celery cut small
    One half cup of corn (whole)

Stir and set aside.

Sauce: Place the following in a Vitamix or blender

    Three tablespoons of hot sauce
    One half cup of whole wheat sifted pastry flour
    One teaspoon of onion powder
    One teaspoon of maple syrup
    Twelve ounces of cooked rice
    One half teaspoon of bio-salt
    One and half cups of water
    One fourth of teaspoon of marjoram
    One fourth cup of Braggs amino
    One stalk of celery
    One half teaspoon of thyme
    One teaspoonful of garlic powder
    One fourth teaspoon of dill weed
    One teaspoon of basil
    Three tablespoon of corn meal
    One fourth teaspoon of savory
    One fourth teaspoon of sage

Add all of the ingredients above to a large pan. Stir and add twelve ounces of red or pinto beans (cooked) and four large baked potatoes cut and peeled in a pan.

Crust: Place the following in a Vitamix or blender:

One cup of ground almonds
One cup of oatmeal flour
One fourth cup of coconut

Then pour ingredients into a bowl and add for tablespoons of water and mix

This recipe makes thirteen hot pies, if using a seven inch baking dishes

Form dough into crust, in the baking dishes.

Bake crust for ten minutes at 350 degrees, and then add the ingredients to the shell. With the same crust sprinkle crumbs to form a top crust and return to the oven at 350 degrees for 30 minutes.

Recipe 95 ——————————————————

Basic Cookies with Frosting

Place the following in a Vitamix or blender:

    Two thirds cup of almond butter
    One fourth cup of tofu
    One half cup of sucanant sugar
    One fourth teaspoon of bio-salt

Pour into a bowl and add one and three fourths cup of whole wheat pastry flour sifted.

Mix and roll and use a cookie cutter.

Place on cookie tray lined with parchment paper or a cookie mat.

Bake at 400 degrees for 6-8 minutes

Let cool.

For the frosting see Any Doughnut Toppings or in a small bowl mix:

    Two tablespoonfuls of soymilk
    One cup of sucanant sugar

Add to cookies and sprinkle with coconut flour on top.

Recipe 96

Baking Taco Shells

Place corn tortillas on the grill directly folded over to form a taco shell

Two wires should separate the two ends. Bake for 5-8 minutes on 350 degrees

When baked; can add beans, lettuce, avocado, onion, and sauce

Recipe 97 ——————————————————

Any Fruit Pastry

Crust:

Place the following in a large bowl:

>   Two cups of maple syrup
>   Two cups of almond butter
>   Two cups of whole wheat pastry flour sifted
>   Two cups of almonds (chopped)

Mix and place on a cookie tray lined with parchment paper. Dough will be sticky, so pat down with back side of spoon. Do not use a flat cookie tray use cookie tray with edges.

Bake at 350 degrees for 25 minutes.

Filling:

Place the following in a Vitamix or blender:

>   One brick of tofu (or one pound)
>   Two teaspoons of lemon juice
>   Two cups of maple syrup
>   Two cups of any fruit

Then place on top of cooked dough.

Then add one and one half cups of chopped almonds.

Bake ten to twelve minutes in oven at 350 degrees

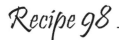 *Recipe 98*

Pineapple Frosting

For five minutes on low, place the following in a pan:

   Three fourths cup of pineapple juice
   Three tablespoons of tapioca
   One fourth teaspoon of bio-salt
   One fourth teaspoon of vanilla

Then place in a Vitamix or blender.

Then pour in a bowl and add three fourths cup of coconut. This is not sweet, to be used as decoration only. See Any Doughnut Topping Recipe, place pineapple frosting on top.

Recipe 99 ————————————————

Pineapple Upside-down Cake

Sprinkle with one cup of sucanant sugar inside the pan, lined with parchment paper then add one half cup of maple syrup.

Add five slices of pineapple rings, and use 15 cherries, Bing or Queen Ann.

Put five cherries in the center of the pineapples.

Then put the other cherries anywhere, set aside

Dough:

Place the following in a Vitamix or blender:

    Two cups of almond butter
    Twelve tablespoons of pineapple juice
    Two cups of maple syrup
    Six cups of whole wheat pastry flour sifted

If the blender is not powerful enough, place the mixed ingredients in a bowl and stir.

Let sit at room temperature then add

    Two tablespoons of yeast in ¼ cup of finger warm water

Let sit for two hours or until dough rises

Mix and pour into cake pan

Bake at 350 degrees for 45 minutes. Use toothpick test to see if center is done.

Let cool for one hour or more. Place plate on top of cake pan and turn over, then carefully remove the parchment paper.

Recipe 100

Hot Beans for Burritos

In a large pan soak overnight:

> Five cups of pinto or red beans

And add water 4-5 inches above beans.

The next day boil for ten minutes.

Change water and add raw potato and continue to boil, and then turn to low

Then add:

> Two tablespoons of chili powder
> Two tablespoons of paprika
> One tablespoon of garlic powder
> One tablespoon of bio-salt
> One tablespoon of maple syrup
> Two teaspoons of cayenne pepper
> One half onions (chopped)
> Two cups of chopped peppers or one cup of crushed red peppers.

Boil for two hours or until water is gone.

Do not eat the potato, remove and discard.

Recipe 101

Apricot Pie

See Special Pie Crust No. 38

Place into an uncooked pie shell two pounds of apricots cut small.

Place the following into a Vitamix or blender and add another two pounds of apricots (minus pits)

Then pour this into a pan with one fourth teaspoon of bio-salt.

    One cup of maple syrup
    One cup of sucanant sugar

Then add three tablespoons of tapioca

Boil for 30 minutes more on warm and stir.

Pour into pie shell and bake for 45 minutes at 350 degrees.

For a very firm filling boil 30 minutes longer.

Recipe 102

Apple Pie

See Special Pie Crust Recipe No. 38

Place into uncooked pie shell, two cups of cut and peeled apples (bite size) and set aside.

Then place the following in a Vitamix or blender:

The above apple feelings, two to three apples (cored)
Add one cup of water

Pour into a pan and add the following:

One cup of maple syrup
One cup of sucanant sugar
One fourth teaspoon of bio-salt
One tablespoonful of cinnamon

Boil one and half four on warm, and then add three tablespoons of tapioca and boil for another half hour on warm. Pour sauce in pie shell and bake for 45 minutes at 350 degrees.

For a very firm filling boil 30 minutes longer.

Recipe 103 _____

Plum Pie

See Special Pie Crust No 38

Place into uncooked pie shell two pounds of plums cut small

Place in a Vitamix or blender another two pounds of plums (minus pits)

Then pour this into a pan with one fourth teaspoon of bio-salt

　　One cup of maple syrup
　　One cup of sucanant sugar

Boil one and half hours on warm

Then add three tablespoons of tapioca flour

Boil for 30 minutes more on warm and stir. Pour into a pie shell and bake for 45 minutes at 350 degrees.

For a very firm filling boil 30 minutes longer.

Recipe 104

Pizza Sauce No. 3

Place the following in a pan and boil for two hours:

> One half cup of almond butter
> Two teaspoons of oregano
> Two teaspoons of marjoram
> One onion cut small
> Two teaspoons of bio-salt
> One can of olives cut each on one half
> Twenty tomatoes cut small
> One tablespoon of maple syrup
> Four cloves of garlic cut small

Add six cups of water only.

Sauce must be thick boil longer if needed. Freeze extra in 12 ounce cups

Recipe 105

Pizza Sauce No. 1

Place the following into a pan and boil for two hours until thick:

Three teaspoons of almond butter
Two onions chopped small
Three cloves of garlic cut small
Twenty tomatoes cut small
One can of olives cut each in half
Three teaspoons of thyme
Three teaspoons of basil
Three teaspoons of parsley
Three teaspoons of maple syrup
Three teaspoons of oregano
Two teaspoons of bio-salt

Add six cups of water.

Sauce must be thick. Continue to boil if needed place extra in 12 ounce cups and freeze.

Recipe 106

COFFEE MUFFINS

Place in a vitamix all of the following:

Three fourths cup of soymilk
One half teaspoon of Biosalt
4 Tablespoons of Almond butter
4 Tablespoons of Sucanant sugar
One fourth Cup of Tofu

Mix and pour into a bowl and add the following:

2 Tablespoons of roma
One and three fourths cups of Whole wheat pastry flour (sifted)
1 Tablespoon of yeast (mix into one fourth cup finger warm water, let sit for 2 hours, dough should rise.

Mix and place into cup cake holders and place into muffin pans.

Bake 400 degrees for 10-15 minutes.

Use toothpick test after 10 minutes to see if center is baked.

Can add frosting when cool

Recipe 107 _____

Gloria Duggins Pecan Candy

Boil the following on warm for thirty minutes:

Six cups of maple syrup
Three tablespoon of soy milk
One a half teaspoons of bio-salt
Six tablespoons of almond butter
Three cups of grinded walnuts

Boil for fifteen minutes on warm. Then add:

Two tablespoons of carob
Two tablespoons of roma

Boil for fifteen more minutes.

Add three cups of puffed rice and boil for fifteen more minutes. Stir

until thick. Pour on to parchment paper. Add another layer of parchment paper

on top of ingredients and then will rolling pin, roll thin. Let cool and cut.

Recipe 108

Pete Panagopoulos Almond Fudge

In a pan boil the following on warm for five minutes:

> One cup of maple syrup
> Two and a half cups of sucanant sugar

Continue to boil on warm for another five minutes and add the following:

> One tablespoon of roma
> One tablespoon of carob

Boil on warm for five more minutes and add two cups of almonds (ground)

Boil on warm for five more minutes and add two and a half cups of almond butter.

Continue to boil on warm for five more minutes and stir.

Then our into a glass dish, lined with parchment paper

Let cool and cut into squares.

Recipe 109

Pete & Rosa Cerrillo Cinnamon Walnut Candy

In a large pan boil the following for ten minutes on warm:

Four teaspoons of cinnamon
One cup of maple syrup
Two and a half cups of sucanant sugar

Then add:

Two cups of chopped walnuts

Boil for ten more minutes on warm. Add:

Two and a half cups of almond butter and boil for five more minutes on warm.

Continue to stir until thick.

Then place into mold or cup cake holders, can use parchment paper, or rubber mold.

Let cool before removing from the mold.

Keep refrigerated

Recipe 110 —————————————————————————

Sugared Nuts

In a large bowl mix one cup of the following:

    Walnuts, pecans, almonds, hazel nuts, Brazil nuts, and maple syrup

For example, if Brazil nut is not available substitute with one of the other nuts

Mix and then add one teaspoon of bio-salt and two cups of sucanant sugar

Mix and place on a cookie tray lined with parchment paper.

Turn the oven to 200 degrees and continue to bake for 12 hours or overnight

Bake until mixture is dry.

Do not double recipe.

Recipe 111 _____

Papaya Candy

Mix the following in a large bowl:

Eight tablespoons of wheat germ
Two teaspoons of bio-salt
Six cups of maple syrup
Two teaspoons of vanilla
Four teaspoons of flaxseed meal
Two cups of chopped walnuts
Twelve cups of dry papaya cut small

Mix and add:

Four cups of oatmeal flour
Four cups of whole wheat pastry flour sifted

Mix and place into a glass dish 9x13 inches lined with parchment paper.

Bake at 200 degrees for two and a half hours.

Let cool. Place in a refrigerator for twenty four hours and cut into Squares

Recipe 112

Carob Cake

Mix the following in a large bowl:

    Six cups of maple syrup
    Two tablespoons of almond butter
    One tablespoon of bio-salt
    Four tablespoons of carob
    Four tablespoons of roma
    Two tablespoons of rosewater
    One teaspoon of vanilla
    Six cups of grounded walnuts

Mix and add:

    Four cups of sifted whole wheat pastry flour

Mix and place all the ingredients in a 9x13 inch glass dish lined with parchment paper. Bake at 350 degrees for fifty minutes. Use the toothpick test to see if center of the cake is cooked, if not check every five minutes until toothpick is cleaned. Let cool and cut into desired pieces.

Recipe 113 ────────────────

Thelma Main Hazel Nut Fudge

In a pan boil the following on warm for five minutes:

    One cup of maple syrup
    Two and a half cups of sucanant sugar

Boil on warm for five more minutes and add the following:

    One tablespoon of roma
    One tablespoon of carob

Boil on warm for five more minutes and add two cups of hazelnuts (chopped).

Boil on warm for five more minutes and add two and a half cups of almond butter

Continue to boil on warm for five minutes and stir. Then pour into a glass dish, lined with parchment paper. Let cool and cut into squares.

Recipe 114

CORN MEAL AND WHEAT PIZZA

Place in a large bowl the following:

    1 Cup of sifted whole wheat pastry flour
    Three fourths cup of cornmeal
    2 teaspoons of Biosalt

Mix and add:

    3 tablespoons of water
    One and one fourth cup of almond butter

Continue to mix, this is a crumb crust, form into small oven bowls (4 x 4 inch only)

Bake using parchment paper lined bowls.

Bake 375 degrees for 15 minutes.

Helpful hint: Before placing in oven let set in refrigerator for 20 minutes

Recipe 115 ———————————————————————————————

Margaret & Harvey Binder Pecan Fudge

In a pan boil the following for five minutes on warm:

    One cup of maple syrup
    Two and a half cups of sucanant sugar
    Boil on warm for five more minutes and add the following:
    One tablespoon of roma
    One tablespoon of carob

Boil on warm for five more minutes and add two cups of pecans (ground).

Boil on warm for five more minutes and add two and a half cups of almond butter

Continue to boil on warm for five more minutes and stir. Then pour into a glass dish, lined with parchment paper. Let cool and cut into squares.

Recipe 116

Michael F Mooney Pecan Roma Carob Candy

Boil on warm in a large pan the following for thirty minutes:

> six cups of maple syrup
> Three tablespoon of soy milk
> Six tablespoons of almond butter
> One and a half teaspoon of bio-salt

Add two teaspoons of carob powder and two teaspoons of roma.

Boil for fifteen more minutes on warm and stir, and add three cups of pecans (ground). Boil for fifteen more minutes on warm and continue to stir. And three cups of puffed rice. Boil for fifteen more minutes and continue to stir. When thick, pour on to parchment paper.

Add another layer of parchment paper on top of the ingredients and then with a rolling pin, roll thin.

Let cool and cut.

Recipe 117 —————————————————————————————

Bell Huck Walnut Fudge

In a pan boil the following on warm for five minutes:

> One cup of maple syrup
> Two and a half cups of sucanant sugar

Boil on warm for five more minutes and add the following:

> One tablespoon of roma
> One tablespoon of carob

Boil on warm for five more minutes and add two cups of walnuts (ground).

Boil on warm for five more minutes and add two and a half cups of almond butter

Continue to boil on warm for five more minutes and stir. Then pour into a glass dish, lined with parchment paper. Let cool and cut into squares.

Recipe 118 _____

Sauce for the inside of Cinnamon Rolls

In a large pan place the following:

    Twenty two cups of maple syrup

    Three teaspoons of bio-salt

    Eight teaspoons of vanilla

    Eight teaspoons of rose water

    Twenty tablespoons of cinnamon

    Four cups of almond butter

    Eight tablespoons of soy milk

    Eight cups of roasted walnuts

Boil for 45 minutes on low. Then add four tablespoons of tapioca flour.

Then boil on low for fifteen more minutes then turn to warm until sauce is thick

Place the warm sauce on dough; do not put this sauce on top of rolls, for inside only.

Can make in advance, place in refrigerator.

Recipe 119 —————————————————

Nectarine Pie

See Special Pie Crust Recipe #38

Place in an uncooked pie crust: Two pounds of cut-small-peeled nectarines.

Set aside in a cool place.

Place into a Vitamix, two more pounds of nectarines and the peelings from above. Then pour into a pan and add the following:

> One fourth teaspoon of bio-salt
> One cup of maple syrup
> One cup of sucanant sugar

Boil for one a half hours on warm.

Then add:

> Three tablespoons of tapioca

Boil for thirty more minutes on warm.

Pour the sauce into pie crust.

Bake at 350 degrees for 45 minutes.

For a very firm filling, boil 30 minutes longer.

Recipe 120

Cookies Carob Plain or Roma

Place the following in a Vitamix or blender:

> Two cups of almond butter
> One and one-half cups of maple syrup
> One fourth cup of tofu
> One fourth teaspoon of bio-salt
> One teaspoon of vanilla
> One half teaspoon of peppermint water

Then add in a bowl: the above and

> Two and two thirds cups of whole wheat pastry flour sifted

For carob cookies add one half cup of carob powder.

For roma cookies add one half cup of roma.

Mix the above together. Use cookie tray lined with parchment paper or a cookie matt.

Form cookies on the tray.

Bake for 8-10 minutes at 350 degrees.

Recipe 121 ———————————————————

Carob Pastry

Place the following in a large bowl:

    One and one fourth cups of whole wheat pastry flour sifted
    One cup of maple syrup
    One fourth cup of roma and one fourth cup of carob powder
    One cup of almond butter

Mix and place in 8 x 8 glass baking dish lined parchment paper.

Bake at 350 degrees for 15 minutes.

Place the following in a Vitamix:

    Three cups of soy milk
    One fourth cup of tofu
    Two teaspoons of vanilla

Mix and add:

    One and a half cup of chopped pecans and
    Add to the above crust

Return to oven. Bake at 350 degrees for 20-25 minutes.

Let cool and cut into bars.

Recipe 122

Spice Butter Cookies

Add the following to a Vitamix or blender:

    One and a half teaspoons of cinnamon
    Three teaspoons of vanilla
    Two and a half cups of maple syrup
    Three cups of almond butter
    One teaspoon of bio-salt

Pour into a large bowl and add:

    Four cups of whole wheat pastry flour sifted

Mix and roll and use a cookie cutter for shape and place on tray lined with parchment paper or cookie matt.

Bake at 350 degrees for ten minutes.

Recipe 123 _____

Oatmeal Crackers

In a Vitamix or blender, add the following:

> One cup of water
> One cup of oatmeal
> One half teaspoon of bio-salt

Pour batter on cookie sheet and sprinkle poppy seeds and sesame seeds on top of batter.

Batter is very thick, so spread on cookie tray thin with plastic knife. May require two trays. This depends on how thick you want your crackers.

Bake at 350 degrees for 10 minutes and remove tray from the oven and with a plastic knife cut into squares.

Return to oven for 20 minutes until crisp.

*Recipe 124*_____

Cinnamon Sugar Doughnut Topping

For top of doughnuts:

    In a small bowl mix the following:
    One half cup of sucanant sugar
    One tablespoon of cinnamon
    One half cup of maple syrup Or:
    One cup of sucanant sugar
    One tablespoon of cinnamon

Roll on both sides of the doughnuts in a bag.

Recipe 125 ⎯⎯⎯⎯⎯⎯⎯⎯⎯⎯⎯⎯⎯⎯⎯⎯

Jelly Doughnuts

Filling for inside of doughnut

In a Vitamix or blender mix the following:

    One and one fourth cups of fruit with one fourth cup of maple syrup

Or see Any Fruit Pie Recipe for jam-like filling

Recipe 126

Strudel Dough

Place the following in a Vitamix or blender:

> One cup of almond butter
> One fourth cup of tofu
> One cup of warm water

In a large bowl, pour the above and add one half teaspoon of bio-salt; add three cups of sifted whole wheat pastry flour.

Mix all of the above and knead on a cookie matt for five minutes or more.

Roll into four balls and then roll each ball into a square by using a rolling pin. In the center of the square place two tablespoons almond butter on the center of the dough. Then place fruit two to three inches from the side of the square. Pour sucanant sugar over the fruit and add one spoon of chopped walnuts on top of the fruit.

(For Fruit see Special Pie Recipes)

Roll and cut into squares, place on cookie tray lined with parchment paper or a cookie matt.

Bake at 350 degrees for 30 minutes.

Recipe 127 —————————————————————

Date Cup Cookie

The night before, place the following in a large bowl:

> Four cups of dates
> One fourth teaspoon of bio-salt
> One teaspoon of vanilla
> One half cup of sucanant sugar

Mix. Cover the bowl and place in refrigerator. The next day place bowl in microwave oven to soften. Then pour into Vitamix or blender and make into sauce paste.

The Dough: The night before make dough (see Recipe 45 Butter Cookie Recipe)

Then cover bowl and place in refrigerator covered.

The next day roll out dough and cut into circle. (Approximate cookie size 4x4inches). Place two spoons of date mixture inside the circle, then place one tablespoon of ground walnuts on top of date mixture.

Place in paper cup cake holders, then place in muffin pan. Do not press dough into cup cake holders because it will stick.

Place in oven and bake at 375 degrees for 20-25 minutes.

Recipe 128

Italian Sauce

Place the following in a Vitamix or blender:

    One half teaspoon of marjoram
    Four cloves of garlic
    Two teaspoons of bio-salt
    Twenty two tomatoes
    Eight cups of water only
    Two tablespoons of oregano
    Two tablespoons of Italian seasoning

Blend until smooth, then pour into a large pan and add the following:

    Two carrots shredded
    One stalk of celery cut small
    Two bell peppers
    One onion cut small
    One can of olives each cut in half

Boil for two hours on low. Pour on cookies pasta.

Recipe 129

Lasagna

Boil for ten minutes on high, one pound of 16 ounces of lasagna (do this last)

Place in a pan the following and boil for two hours on low:

    One tablespoon of bio-salt
    Twenty tomatoes cut small
    Two bell peppers cut small
    One can of olives cut each in half
    Two carrots shredded
    One onion cut small

Then combine 6-12 ounce cups of one of the following recipes:

    Spanish 145; Italian 128; Tagliatetle 157; or Tomato Sauce 153

Then in a glass dish 13x9 inches, place one to three cups of sauce on bottom of glass dish, then cover dish with one layer of noodles and place enough sauce. And repeat process and bake for thirty minutes at 350 degrees

Recipe 130

Bob Panagopoulos Pizza Sauce No. 2

In a Vitamix or blender, place the following:

    Twenty tomatoes

    Three teaspoons of maple syrup

    One teaspoon of bio-salt

    Two teaspoons of oregano

    Four cloves of garlic

    Four teaspoons of almond butter

    Six cups of water

Then pour into a large pan and add the following:

    One onion cut small

    One can of olives cut each into one half

    One bell pepper cut small

Continue to boil two hours on low.

Sauce must be thick.

Place sauce as desired on baked pasta shell and warm when ready to serve

Can freeze extra in 12 ounce cups

Recipe 131

Cuban Black Beans in Rice

Place in a pan and boil the following until mixture is thick:

    Six tomatoes chopped
    One onion chopped
    One stalk of celery chopped
    One bell pepper chopped
    Two tablespoons of Braggs-Ammino
    One teaspoon of parsley
    Two tablespoons of lemon juice
    One half teaspoon of turmeric powder
    One teaspoon of bio-salt
    Two teaspoons of chili powder

Continue to boil between five to ten minutes on low until mixture is thick

Then add six ounces of cooked black beans. Add to cooked rice and mix.

Recipe 132

Black Beans

The night before, place two cups of black beans in a pan. Place enough water to cover three to four inches above the beans. The next day, bring the beans to a boil for ten minutes. Then replace the water.

Then bring to a boil again and add the following:

> One clean raw potato (this will soak up some of the acid)
> One teaspoon of bio-salt
> One teaspoon of garlic powder
> One teaspoon of paprika
> One teaspoon of maple syrup

Continue to boil for two hours or more on low. Use lid to cover the pan.

Check and stir occasionally.

Recipe 133

Light Fudge

In a pan, boil the following for five minutes:

> One cup of maple syrup
> Two and a half cups of sucanant sugar

Boil on warm for five or more minutes and add:

> Two and a half cups of almond butter

Continue to stir and boil another five minutes, until thick. Place in a glass dish (8x8 inches) lined with parchment paper. Let cool, then refrigerate for an hour or more and cut into squares

Recipe 134

Dark Fudge

Place the following in a pan:

> One cup of maple syrup
> Two and a half cups of sucanant sugar

Boil on warm for five minutes.

Then place one tablespoon of carob and one tablespoon of roma in a pan and stir. Boil for five minutes more on warm.

Then place in a pan two and a half cups of almond butter and continue to boil on warm. Continue to stir for two to five minutes on warm. Then place in a glass dish (approximately 8x8inches) lined with parchment paper.

Let cool and refrigerate.

When cool cut into squares.

Recipe 135

Pigeon Beans

In a large pan, soak the following the night before:

One pound of pigeon beans.

The next day boil for ten minutes and replace the water. Add eight cups of water and one clean potato. This will absorb some of the acid. Boil until soft.

Cover with lid.

After beans are cooked, throw the potato away.

Recipe 136

Pigeon Rice

The night before in a large pan place the following:

> Eight cups of water
> Six cups of rice
> One teaspoon of bio-salt

Then next day boil for ten to fifteen minutes and cover with a lid.

Then add to cooked rice:

> Twelve ounces of pigeon beans
> One tablespoon of bio-salt
> One teaspoon of thyme
> One teaspoon of onion powder
> One teaspoon of garlic powder

The stir into rice mixture, Return lid to pan and let sit for an hour. Turn heat off. Place in 6-12 ounce cups.

Can freeze extra

Recipe 137

Alexander Panagopoulos Sweet and Sour Sauce No. 1

Boil the following in a pan:

> Four and a half cups of water
> Two cups of lemon juice
> Eight teaspoons of whole wheat pastry flour sifted
> One and one third cup of maple syrup
> Twelve tablespoons of tomato paste.

Continue to boil and stir until thick.

Can freeze extra

*Recipe 138*_____

Inez Speidell Sweet and Sour Sauce No. 2

Boil the following in a pan:

Two tablespoon of almond butter

Three tablespoons of ginger

One and half tablespoons of whole wheat pastry flour sifted

Two and half cups of water

Four tablespoons of lemon juice

Three tablespoons of tomato paste

One half cup of maple syrup

Three tablespoons of Braggs-Ammino

Boil on low and continue to stir until thick.

Can freeze extra

Recipe 139

Very Very Hot Sauce

Place the following in a Vita mix or blender:

> Two tablespoon of garlic powder or five cloves of garlic
> One cup of maple syrup
> Two tablespoons of onion powder or one onion (place in blender)
> Four cups of red crushed peppers, or
> Two cups of cayenne or two cups of red crushed peppers.
> Two teaspoons of cumin
> Two tablespoons of bio-salt
> One cup of lemon juice

Place in a blender:

> One half cup of cilantro
> 26 tomatoes or 26 cups of tomatoes and two cups of fresh peppers
> Five to six cups of water

Then pour into pan.

Boil for two hours or more until thick.

Can freeze extra until ready to serve

Recipe 140

Lentils

In a pan boil on low the following for thirty minutes or more:

    Add seven cups of water
    One pound of dry lentils
    One half onions cut small or one tablespoon of onion powder
    One tablespoon of garlic powder
    One stalk of celery cut small
    One tablespoon of bio-salt

One tablespoon of parsley

Do not soak lentils over night. Cover with lid.

Follow the instructions on the package for cooking instructions.

Recipe 141 _____

Shrimp Sauce

Place the following into a Vita Mix or blender:

> One teaspoon of clove powder
> Two tablespoons of Braggs-Ammino
> Two tablespoons of garlic powder (or five cloves of garlic)
> 18 tomatoes or 18 cups of tomatoes
> Two cups of lemon juice
> Three tablespoons of Cayenne Pepper
> Two tablespoons of onion powder
> Two tablespoons of bio-salt
> One tablespoon of chili powder
> Two teaspoons of dill weed
> One cup of maple syrup
> Four to six cups of water

Boil for two hours or until sauce is thick

Can freeze extra until needed

Recipe 142

Almond Carob Candy

In a large pan place the following:

    Six cups of maple syrup
    Three tablespoons of soy milk
    One and a half teaspoons of bio-salt
    Six tablespoons of almond butter

Boil on warm for thirty minutes. Stir occasionally.

Add three cups of almonds (ground or chopped)

Boil for fifteen minutes on warm and four teaspoons of carob powder.

Boil for fifteen minutes on warm, and add three cups of puffed rice.

Continue to stir. Boil for fifteen more minutes on low until mixture is thicker than oatmeal consistency.

Pour mixture on parchment paper and then place another sheet of parchment paper over this and roll thin with a rolling pin.

Let cool and break into squares.

Place extra in refrigerator

Recipe 143

Carob Roma Candy

In a large pan, boil the following on warm for thirty minutes:

Six tablespoons of almond butter
Six cups of maple syrup
Three tablespoons of soy milk
One and a half teaspoons of bio-salt

Then add three cups of puffed rice and boil fifteen minutes on warm and then add:

Two teaspoons of roma
Two teaspoons of carob

Then boil fifteen minutes on warm and stir, then add:

Three more cups of puffed rice

Boil for fifteen more minutes on warm and stir until very tick. Place mixture on parchment paper, two sheets side by side. Then cover mixture with two more sheets of parchment paper. Then roll thin using a rolling pin. Let cool and break into desired shaped.

*Recipe 144*_____

WALNUT CINNAMON CLUSTERS

In a large pan on warm boil the following:

    6 Cups of maple syrup
    3 tablespoons of soymilk
    6 tablespoons of almond butter
    One and a half teaspoons of Biosalt

Add and boil for 15 minutes on warm:

    3 Cups of grinded walnuts

Add and boil for 15 minutes on warm:

    4 teaspoons of cinnamon

Add and boil on low for 15 minutes:

    3 cups of Puffed Rice

Continue to stir until thick.

On a countertop place 2 large pieces of parchment paper side by side. Pour mixture from pan on top of parchment paper, and then place 2 more pieces of parchment paper on top of mixture. Then with a rolling pin, roll thin.

Let cool and break into desired pieces.

Recipe 145 ————————————————————————————

TAMARA NEUMILLER SPANISH PASTA

In a vitamix, place the following:

    11 whole tomatoes
    8 cups of water

Then pour into a large pan with the following:

    11 diced tomatoes
    2 diced onions
    8 cloves of diced garlic
    ¼ cup paprika
    ¼ cup chili powder
    2 tablespoons dried parsley
    1 tablespoon of maple syrup
    1 tablespoon of Biosalt
    1 can of olives, cut in halves

Boil for 1 hour and 40 minutes on low heat

In a second pan boil two pounds of pasta:

(follow your instructions on pasta wrapper)

Then empty pan of water and add enough sauce to cover pasta, stir and boil for twenty minutes on low heat. Stir frequently to prevent pasta from sticking to pan.

Recipe 146

CHINESE RICE

Boil in a pan the following:

    One half cup of olives cut each in half
    1 large onion cut small
    2 Bell Peppers cut small
    One half stalk of celery cut small
    One and one half cups of green peas
    1 Tablespoonful of Paprika
    4 Tablespoonfuls of Braggs Ammino
    1 Teaspoonful of Basil
    1 Teaspoonful of Biosalt

Continue to boil for 10 to 20 minutes on low. Add to cooked rice and mix.

Recipe 147

CHILI BEANS - PINTO OR RED

The night before, place in a large pan 5 cups of dry beans. Then add enough water to cover, 3 to 4 inches above the beans.

The next day bring to a boil for 10 minutes, and then replace the water adding water again.

Place on stove top and bring to a boil, then turn to low. Add a clean potato, this soaks up some of the acid.

Add the following:

Ingredients:

    1 Teaspoon of Lemon Juice
    1 Onion cut small
    4 Cloves of Garlic cut small
    2 Bell Peppers
    10 Tomatoes or Ten Cups of Tomatoes
    2 Tablespoons of Braggs Amino
    2 Tablespoons of Biosalt
    1 Teaspoon of Maple Syrup

Directions:

Continue to boil until water is gone. (Remove the potato and throw away)

Recipe 148

TAMALES

First boil on low 2 cups of Flaxseed meal -- boil in 2 cups of water for one half hour, stir and then add to the bowls.

Divide the following into 2 large bowls:

11 and a half cups of yellow corn meal flour
14 cups of Water
2 Tablespoonfuls of Biosalt
2 Cups of frozen corn
1 Cup of Sesame seeds
2 Cups of Blue corn meal or one half pound
2 Cups of corn meal

Mix and set aside.

For the inside of tamales boil on low for 1-2 hours the following:

1 Tablespoonful of Maple syrup
10 tomatoes cut small
2 Bell peppers cut small
1 Onion cut small
2 Cups of whole corn
2 Teaspoonfuls of Dill
4 Teaspoonfuls of Cumin
1 Teaspoonful of Biosalt
2 Teaspoonfuls of Paprika
2 Teaspoonfuls of Chili Powder
2 Tablespoonfuls of Garlic Powder
3 Cans of olives cut each in one half

Continue to boil, sauce must be thick.

Notes: make day before & cool & stored in tightly covered bowl to save time.

To prepare the corn husks, boil on low for 3 to 5 minutes, and then place corn mixture into the husk. Then place enough sauce in center and wrap. Make sure at least 2 to 4 olives in each. In a large pan place wrapped tamales upright with 3 to 4 inches of water.

Boil for 45 minutes on low, or until cooked.

Recipe 149

VEGETABLE SOUP

Boil in a large pan the following:

>   17 Cups of Water
>   1 Cup of Bob's Red Mill Veggie Mix
>   2 Tablespoonfuls of Braggs Ammino
>   One half teaspoonful of Chili Powder
>   1 Teaspoonful of Biosalt
>   One half teaspoonful of Paprika

Boil for 2 hours on low.

Can freeze extra

Recipe 150

CAROB ROMA COOKIE

Place in a large bowl the following:

> One half cup of Almond Butter, and 2 tablespoonfuls of Almond Butter
> One fourth cup of Tofu
> Three fourths cup of chopped walnuts
> One half cup of Roma
> One half cup of Carob
> 1 teaspoonful of Vanilla

Roll out the dough on a cookie matt and use cookie cutter shape as desired.

Bake at 375 degrees for 10 to 12 minutes.

This is not sweet. Dough,

This requires a frosting on top; also see frosting recipe No. 23.

Recipe 151

Ray & Linda Panagopoulos
SUNFLOWER SEED AND COCONUT WAFFLES

Place in a vitamix or blender the following:

> 1 Cup of Sunflower seeds
> One and a half cups of Oatmeal
> 1 Cup of Corn meal
> One half teaspoonful of Biosalt
> 3 and half cups of Water
> One half cup of Coconut

Pour into a hot waffle iron.

Bake for 13 to 15 minutes. Serve hot.

Can freeze extra

Recipe 152

WAFFLES OATMEAL AND ALMOND

Place in a vitamix or blender the following:

2 1/2 cups of Water......or 2 and a half cups of Soymilk
1 & 1/2 cups of Oatmeal
One fourth cup of Sunflower seeds
One third cup of Almonds
One half teaspoonful of Biosalt

Pour into a hot waffle iron. Bake for 13 to 15 minutes.

Serve hot.

Can freeze extra

Recipe 153 ———————————————————

RHI CAROB AND ROMA, COCONUT, OATMEAL, WHOLE WHEAT PASTRY FLOUR COOKIES

Mix the following in a large bowl:

> 6 cups of maple syrup
> 1 teaspoonful of Biosalt
> 1/2 cup of carob
> 1/2 cup of roma

Mix and add 8.8 ounces of lite coconut

> And add 4 cups of oatmeal flour.

Mix and add 5 cups of sifted whole wheat pastry flour.

Form on cookie trays lined with parchment paper or cookie matt.

Bake 325 degrees for 25 minutes.

Recipe 154

HOT SAUCE

place in a vitamix or blender the following

    28 tomatoes
    8 teaspoonfuls of lemon juice
    1 teaspoonful of maple syrup
    add one cup of the following
    crushed red peppers
    cayenne peppers
    jalapeno peppers
    add 6 cups of water.

boil for two hours until sauce is thick.

can freeze extra

Recipe 155

RED BEANS FOR TOP OF RICE

soak overnight in a large pan:

> 2 cups of beans
> enough water to cover, two or more inches above the beans

the next day, boil for ten minutes, then change the water.

Add ten cups of water and the following:

> 1 teaspoonful of Biosalt
> 1 teaspoonful of parsley
> 1 teaspoonful of maple syrup
> 1 teaspoonful of garlic powder
> 1 teaspoonful of paprika

bring to a boil then turn to low. in a vitamix or blender:

add the following:

> 1 cup of water.
> one carrot
> one stalk of celery
> one bell pepper

pour into the above pan and continue to boil until cooked. (add a clean potato, this will absorb some of the acid of beans, after beans are cooked throw potato away)

Recipe 156

CORN MEAL WAFFLES

Place in a vitamix or blender the following:

    5 cups of corn meal (not corn flour)

    6 cups of water

    2 Teaspoonfuls of Biosalt

    1 and one third cups of cleaned Cashews

    1 Tablespoon of Maple syrup

Place in a waffle iron and cook between 13 to 15 minutes.

Can freeze extra

Recipe 157

TAGLIATETLE SAUCE

in a large pan, add the following:

    8 cups of water
    1 teaspoonful of maple syrup
    two onions chapped small
    one stalk of celery chopped small
    two carrots grated
    two bell peppers cut small
    2 teaspoonfuls of chili powder
    1 teaspoonful of marjoram
    four cloves of garlic chopped
    2 teaspoonfuls of Biosalt
    one can of olives cut each in one half
    eleven tomatoes cut small

place an additional eleven tomatoes in vitamix or blender and pour into pan.

boil for one hour and forty minutes on low

then add enough of the sauce to cover two pounds of cooked pasta and continue to boil for twenty more minutes and stir occasionally.

can freeze extra

*Recipe 158*_____

Almond Butter Cookies 1

In a large bowl, mix the following:

    Two cups of almond butter
    One cup of sucanant sugar
    One cup of maple syrup
    One half cup of tofu
    One cup of chopped almonds or walnuts

Mix and then add two and a half cups of sifted whole wheat pastry flour.

On a cooking sheet line with parchment paper or a cookie matt, place dough a spoon at a time and form in circles.

Bake at 375 degrees for 15 minutes.

Recipe 159

MAPLE SYRUP FROSTING

Place in a vitamix or blender the following:

    1 Brick or 1 pound of Tofu
    6 teaspoonfuls of Maple syrup
    One half cup of Almond Butter
    One half teaspoonful of Rosewater

Then pour into a pan and boil for 4 to 6 minutes on warm.

Continue to stir until thick.

Recipe 160

ORANGE GLAZE

In a small pan boil the following:

    One fourth cup of Maple Syrup
    4 Tablespoonfuls of Fresh Orange Juice

Boil on warm, stir for a few minutes.

Let cool.

Recipe 161 _____

RYE PANCAKES

in a vitamix or blender place the following

    1/2 cup of tofu

    2 cups of soymilk

    2 teaspoonfuls of almond butter

    2 teaspoonfuls of sucanant sugar

    1 & 1/4 cups of rye flour

    1/2 teaspoonful of Biosalt

make one recipe at a time, if batter is too thick for motor.

follow the cooking instructions on you pancake unit.

can freeze extra until ready to serve

Recipe 162

PANCAKES

place in a vitamix or blender the following

    2 & 1/2 cups of soymilk
    1/2 cups of tofu
    4 teaspoonfuls of almond butter
    1 teaspoonful of Biosalt
    4 teaspoonfuls of sucanant sugar
    2 cups of whole wheat pastry flour

make one recipe at a time

follow the cooking instructions on your pancake unit

can freeze extra until ready to serve

Recipe 163

BLUEBERRY TOPPING

in a small pan place the following

    2 cups of pineapple juice
    3 cups of blueberries
    1/8 teaspoonful of Biosalt

boil on warm for one hour and thirty minutes

then add two tablespoons of tapioca,

continue to boil on warm and stir

can also be used as a jam or filling

Recipe 164

ROMA ICE CREAM

place in a vitamix or blender the following

  1/2 cup of roma
  1/2 cup of soy milk
  one brick of (or pound) tofu
  1/4 teaspoonful of Biosalt
  2 cups of maple syrup
  1 teaspoonful of almond butter
  2 cups of walnuts
  2 cups of puffed rice

blend until smooth

can place in six ounce cups and freeze until ready to serve.

Recipe 165

LEMON ICE CREAM

Directions:

Place in a vitamix or blender the following:

Ingredients:

One fourth teaspoon of Biosalt
Two cups of Walnuts
One brick or one pound of Tofu
One half cup of Soy Milk
One to two cups of Lemon Juice
One tablespoon of Almond Butter
Two cups of Maple Syrup
Three cups of Puffed Rice

Blend until smooth and freeze. Place in 6 ounce cups and store extra in freezer.

Recipe 166

ORANGE DATE SYRUP

Place all of the following in a vitamix or blender:

Ingredients:

    2 Cups of dates
    1 Cup of water
    6 Ounces of orange juice

Directions:

Blend until soft. Place in refrigerator.

Recipe 167

CAROB FUDGE SAUCE

place all of the following in a vitamix or blender

    4 cups of carob powder
    1 cup of roma powder
    Two cups of maple syrup
    1 teaspoonful of Biosalt
    2 cups of almond butter
    1 & 1/2 teaspoonfuls of rosewater
    2 cups of boiling water

Refrigerate before using this sauce which has many uses

Can freeze extra

*Recipe 168*_____

COCONUT LIME FROSTING

Place in a vitamix or blender the following:

    1 cup of Tofu
    One fourth cup of Maple syrup
    1 Tablespoonful of Lime juice
    1 Teaspoonful of grated Lime peeling

Pour in a bowl the above and one cup of coconut.

Mix and let cool in refrigerator.

Recipe 169

CREAMY FROSTING

Place in vitamix or blender the following:

One fourth cup of maple syrup
One fourth cup of whole wheat pastry flour
One fourth cup of soy milk
One half cup of almond butter
One and half teaspoons of rosewater

For creamy lemon frosting, instead of rosewater add one and a half teaspoons of lemon juice and one outside lemon rind.

For creamy orange frosting, instead of rosewater add one and half teaspoons of orange juice and one outside orange rind

Ingredients to Avoid

Bha-butylated bht hydroytolune

Black Strap Molasses

Caffeine

Calcium Sulfate

Carmel

Carrageen

Disodium Sulfite

Distilled water - (do not use- no minerals)

Edtacalcium disodium

Ethylenediamine

Letracetate

Gum Arabic

Cellulose chatti karaya

Gypsum

Hydroylated lecithin

Monocalcium Satisfactory Phosphate

Hydrolyzed protein

Lactic Acid

Magnesium chlorate

Maltodextrim - white sugar

Magnesium Sterate

Modified food starch

Mono+dislycerides

Mono sodium glutamate

M S G

Multol dextrin

Natural flavor

Nisarl

Non hydroxylated Lecithin

Phosforic acid

Popylgallate

Propylene Glycolalginate

Polysorbate 60, 65, 80
Red Dye 40 - Allura Red AC
Stearic Acid
Sodium Saccharin
Sodium Alginate
Sodium Bicarbonate
Sodium Chloride
Sodium Erythrobate
Sulfur Dioxide
Sugar black paperbicarbonate of soda
Tragacanth Xanthan
Torutein
Vinegar
Yeast flakes

RECIPE LIST

1. BAKED POTATO
2. SALADS
3. PASTA
4. PASTA SAUCE - TOMATO SAUCE
5. BROWN RICE
6. TEXAN RICE
7. BELL PEPPER RICE
8. TOSTADAS
9. POPCORN
10. HOT SAUCE
11. CINDY HUCK BEANS FOR BURRITOS
12. TODD NEUMILLER CHINESE SOUP
13. ALMOND BUTTER
14. PIZZA SAUCE
15. PIZZA DOUGH (FOR PIES)
16. WAFFLES
17. TAMALE CASSEROLE
18. MAPLE SYRUP CAKE
19. PAN - FRIED NOODLES
20. FRUIT ICING
21. CAROB BAKED ALASKA
22. VANILLA CAKE
23. CAROB GLAZE
24. MAPLE OATMEAL CAKE
25. CLOVE COOKIES
26. DONALD W. HUCK COCONUT COOKIES

27. CAROB ROMA OATMEAL COOKIES

28. DEEP - DISH PIZZA

29. COCONUT OATMEAL CAROB ROMA COOKIES

30. COCONUT OATMEAL COOKIES

31. CAROB ROMA COCONUT OATMEAL WHOLE-WHEAT PASTRY FLOUR COOKIES

32. COCONUT OATMEAL WHOLE WHEAT PASTRY FLOUR COOKIES

33. STUFFED BELL PAPPERS

34. MAPLE SYRUP COOKIES

35. CAROB COOKIES

36. CAROB BROWN CAKE

37. ANY FRUIT COOKIES (PEACH, CHERRY, APRICOT)

38. SPECIAL PIE CRUST

39. PUMPKIN PIE

40. PARVIN MALEK CAROB PIE

41. ALMOND BUTTER COOKIES 2

42. CAROB FILLING

43. EVELYN ANN MENZIE OLD-FASHIONED GLAZE

44. PINEAPPLE PIE

45. BUTTER COOKIES

46. SUCANANT COOKIES

47. INEZ A. MENZIE COCONUT COOKIES

48. TURNOVERS

49. GOLDEN MACAROONS

50. ORIENTAL CRUNCH

51. PINEAPPLE CANDY

52. CAROB DOUGHNUTS

53. LEMON DOUGHNUTS

54. GRAIN PIZZA

55. CORNMEAL PIZZA

56. CAROB BROWNIES

57. ROBERT E MENZIE WALNUT PIE

58. APRICOT COCONUT WALNUT SQUARES

59. PISTACHIO SCONES

60. EGG ROLLS

61. ROASTED SALTED NUTS

62. FUDGE CUP COOKIE

63. FUDGE SAUCE

64. PINEAPPLE COOKIES

65. TAMALE BEAN PIE

66. NUT PIE

67. DATE WALNUT COOKIES

68. CARAMELIZED GINGER HAZELNUT TART

69. PAPAYA COOKIES

70. CAJUN MIXED NUTS

71. TACO SALAD SHELLS

72. FOR CAKE-WEDDING STYLE CAKE

73. SPANISH MILLET CASSEROLE

74. ENCHILADAS

75. CAROB PIE

76. NUT BUTTER BALLS

77. SHARAREH SHABAFROOZ GARLIC BREAD SPREAD/BUTTER

78. GLAZED CARROT CAKE

79. WAFFLES WITH CASHEWS AND OATMEAL

80. LEMON PINEAPPLE PIE

81. CORN BREAD

82. MATTHEW F. MOONEY ROAST FOR ANY HOLIDAY

83. SPICE DOUGHNUTS

84. SPANISH RICE

85. PINEAPPLE SANDWICH COOKIE

86. CAROB CUP COOKIE

87. ANY FRUIT CUP COOKIE

88. SETAREH TAIS CAKE

89. CAROB DATE PISTACHIO PASTRY

90. FRUIT CAKE COOKIE

91. BAKED MILLET

92. BISCOTTI

93. MULTIGRAIN CRACKERS

94. POT PIE

95. BASIC COOKIE WITH FROSTING

96. TACO SHELLS

97. ANY FRUIT PASTRY

98. PINEAPPLE FROSTING

99. PINEAPPLE UPSIDE DOWN CAKE

100. HOT BEANS FOR BURRITOS

101. APRICOT PIE

102. APPLE PIE

103. PLUM PIE

104. PIZZA SAUCE NO. 3

105. PIZZA SAUCE NO. 1

106. COFFEE MUFFINS

107. GLORIA DUGGINS PECAN CANDY

108. PETER P. PANAGOPOULOS ALMOND FUDGE

109. PETE/ROSA CERRILLO CINNAMON WALNUT CANDY

110. SUGARED NUTS

111. PAPAYA CANDY

112. CAROB CAKE

113. THELMA MAIN HAZELNUT FUDGE

114. WHEAT CORNMEAL PIZZA

115. MARGARET/HARVEY BINDER PECAN FUDGE

116. MICHAEL F. MOONEY PECAN ROMA CAROB CANDY

117. BELLE HUCK WALNUT FUDGE

118. SAUCE FOR INSIDE CINNAMON ROLLS

119. NECTARINE PIE

120. COOKIES/CAROB PLAIN OR ROMA

121. CAROB BARS

122. SPICE BUTTER COOKIES

123. OAT CRACKERS

124. CINNAMON SUGAR DOUGHNUT TOPPING

125. JELLY DOUGHNUT FILLING

126. STRUDEL DOUGH

127. DATE CUP COOKIE

128. ITALIAN SAUCE

129 LASAGNA

130. BOB PANAGOPOULOS PIZZA SAUCE NO. 2

131. CUBAN BLACK BEANS IN RICE

132. BLACK BEANS

133. LIGHT FUDGE

134. DARK FUDGE

135. PIGEON BEANS

136. XENIA PANAGOPOULOS PIGEON RICE

137. ALEXANDRA PANAGOPOULOS SWEET AND SOUR SAUCE NO. 1

138. INEZ SPEIDELL SWEET AND SOUR SAUCE NO. 2

139. VERY VERY HOT SAUCE

225 APRICOT COOKIE BAR

226 GINGER PANCAKES

227 LEMON PASTRY

228 LEMON SUGAR COOKIES

229 DATE BROWNIES

230 ORIGINAL SALT WATER TAFFY

231 AURA VICTORIA HUCK PEPPERMINT SALT WATER TAFFY

232 LEMON SALT WATER TAFFY

233 VANILLA SALT WATER TAFFY

234 ORANGE SALT WATER TAFFY

235 JACK PANAGOPOULOS ROMA SALT WATER TAFFY

236 ADRIANA CERRILLO PECAN SALT WATER TAFFY

237 ELMER LYLE MENZIE ALMOND SALT WATER TAFFY

238 ASHLEY SPEIDELL WALNUT SALT WATER TAFFY

239 ROSS H. MENZIE CAROB SALT WATER TAFFY

240 COCONUT SALT WATER TAFFY

241 CINAMMON SALT WATER TAFFY

242 GINGER SALT WATER TAFFY

243 GENE KOENIG ENGLISH TOFFEE CANDY

244 LUCILLE GILBERT LEMON CHEESECAKE

245 ORANGE CHEESECAKE

246 ASHER MICHAEL NEUMILLER CAROB CHEESECAKE

247 ALLIE NICOLE BLUMA NEUMILLER CAROB CAKE

248 DR. EDE VANILLA SUGAR CAKE

249 WALNUT SQUARE COOKIES

250 TARA SHABAFROOZ PECAN SQUARE COOKIES

251 ALMOND SQUARE COOKIES

252 MARGRET ANN MENZIE PECAN ROPE COOKIES

253 MASSOOD SHABAFROOZ WALNUT ROPE COOKIES

282   POCKET PIZZA 3

283   POCKET PIZZA 4

284   POCKET PIZZA 2

285   POCKET DATE PASTRY

286   POCKET PLUM PASTRY

287   PLUM CREAM PIE

288   POCKET CAROB PASTRY

289   POCKET ROMA PASTRY

290   POCKET WALNUT PASTRY

291   POCKET APRICOT PASTRY

292   POCKET CHERRY PASTRY

293   POCKET PEACH PASTRY

294   POCKET PINEAPPLE - LEMON PASTRY

295   POCKET PUMPKIN PASTRY

296   POCKET APPLE PASTRY

297   POCKET EGG ROLLS

298   POCKET BEAN BURRITO

299   APRICOT CREAM PIE

300   VERA WAIVSCHIDT CHERRY CREAM PIE

301   PEACH CREAM PIE

302   APPLE CREAM PIE

303   TAHEREH TAHERIAN HAVANERO HOT SAUCE

304   SHAHNAZ SHAINEE HOT AND SPICY PINTO BEANS

305   PAYAM MALEK ZADEH CAROB WHEAT COOKIES

306   RAISIN ICE CREAM

307   TOMATO CASSEROLE

308   RAISIN FACE COOKIE

309   DATE FACE COOKIE

310   PINEAPPLE COCONUT SQUARES

311 ORANGE PINEAPPLE ICE CREAM

312 LEMON PINEAPPLE ICE CREAM

313 ROMA FACE COOKIE

314 CAROB FACE COOKIE

315 PUMPKIN FACE COOKIE

316 PINEAPPLE FACE COOKIE

317 APPLE FACE COOKIE

318 PEACH FACE COOKIE

319 APRICOT FACE COOKIE

320 PLUM FACE COOKIE

321 CHERRY FACE COOKIE

322 WALNUT DOME COOKIES

323 ALMOND DOME COOKIES

324 PECAN DOME COOKIES

325 CAROB DOME COOKIES

326 ROMA DOME COOKIES

327 COFFEE CUP COOKIE

328 RAISIN CUP COOKIE

329 WALNUT CUP COOKIE

330 POCKET PASTA NO. 4

331 POCKET PASTA NO. 2

332 POCKET PASTA NO. 3

333 POCKET PASTA NO. 1

334 BRAZIL NUT CARMEL CANDY

335 HAVANERO BAKED RICE

336 MACADAMA CARMEL CANDY

337 CINNAMON CARMEL CANDY

338 WALNUT CARMEL CANDY

339 COCONUT CARMEL CANDY

340 PECAN CARMEL CANDY

341 PISTACHIO CARMEL CANDY

342 HAZEL NUT CARMEL CANDY

343 CASHEW CARMEL CANDY

344 ROASTED ALMOND CARMEL CANDY

345 LEMON CARMEL CANDY

346 ORANGE CARMEL CANDY

347 CAROB CARMEL CANDY

348 ROMA CARMEL CANDY

349 PEPPERMINT CARMEL CANDY

350 GINGER CARMEL CANDY

351 HERBS & GARLIC BAKED RICE

352 WALNUT & ALMOND FROSTING

353 PINEAPPLE & LEMON GLAZE

354 ROMA TOFU COOKIES

355 CAROB TOFU COOKIES

356 CINNAMON TOFU COOKIES

357 RAISIN TOFU COOKIES

358 APRICOT TOFU COOKIES

359 DATE TOFU COOKIES

360 CRANBERRIE TOFU COOKIES

361 SPICE TOFU COOKIES

362 PAPAYA TOFU COOKIES

363 COCONUT TOFU COOKIES

364 LEMON TOFU COOKIES

365 ORANGE TOFU COOKIES

366 PINEAPPLE TOFU COOKIES

367 BLACK BEAN SOUP

368 LEMON COCONUT COOKIES

369 CHERRY SUGAR COOKIES

370 ORANGE SUGAR COOKIES

371 RAISIN SUGAR COOKIES

372 ROMA SUGAR COOKIES

373 APPLE SUGAR COOKIES

374 CAROB SUGAR COOKIES

375 PEPPERMINT SUGAR COOKIES

376 BLUEBERRY SUGAR COOKIE

377 DATE SUGAR COOKIE

378 PINEAPPLE SUGAR COOKIE

379 PLUM SUGAR COOKIE

380 PEACH SUGAR COOKIE

381 APRICOT SUGAR COOKIE

382 NECTURINE SUGAR COOKIE

383 CRANBERRY SUGAR COOKIE

384 PUMPKIN SUGAR COOKIE

385 COCONUT CAROB CARMEL CANDY

386 COCONUT LEMON CARMEL CANDY

387 COCONUT CINNAMON CARMEL CANDY

388 COCONUT ORANGE CARMEL CANDY

389 COCONUT PEPPERMINT CARMEL CANDY

390 COCONUT ROMA CARMEL CANDY

391 COCONUT GINGER CARMEL CANY

392 DATE OATMEAL COOKIE

393 RAISIN OATMEAL COOKIE

394 WALNUT DATE COOKIE

395 WALNUT LEMON COOKIE

396 WALNUT RAISIN COOKIE

397 WALNUT ORANGE COOKIE

427 ITALIAN SPREAD

428 WALNUT WAFFLES

429 POPPY SEED WAFFLES

430 PUMPKIN SEED WAFFLES

431 CAROB SUCANAT SUGAR COOKIE

432 ROMA SUCANAT SUGAR COOKIE

433 PEPPERMINT SUCANAT SUGAR COOKIE

434 CINNAMON SUCANAT SUGAR COOKIE

435 GINGER SUCANAT SUGAR COOKIE

436 CAROB SUGARED NUTS

437 ROMA SUGARED NUTS

438 PECAN PIE

439 BLUEBERRY CREAM PIE

440 GRAPE PIE

References

Dr Herman Aldercreutz, MD., Chief Physician for Helsinki University, Central Hospital, Finland

Dr Peter Greenwald, MD., Director of Cancer Prevention for the National Cancer Institute.

Dr Richard Adamson, MD., Director of National Cancer Institute of Etiology

Dr Milton G. Crane, MD

Dr John H. Kellogg, MD

Dr R. L. Swank, MD., Proceedings of the Society of Experimental and Biological Medicine

Dr Lorraine Day, MD., Cancer Does Not Scare Me Anymore

Dr Wendell Stanley, MD

Dr Hans Nieper, MD

Lyle Cartwright, MD., University of California, Medical Center at San Diego

Dr Kurt Donsbach, N.D.

Eleanor A. Jacobs, PhD.

Printed in the United States
by Baker & Taylor Publisher Services